THE **21** **UNSPOKEN TRUTHS** ABOUT **MARIJUANA**

Antoine Kanamugire, M.D.

BALBOA.
PRESS
A DIVISION OF HAY HOUSE

Balboa Press books may be ordered through booksellers or by contacting:

Balboa Press
A Division of Hay House
1663 Liberty Drive
Bloomington, IN 47403
www.balboapress.com
1 (877) 407-4847

Print information available on the last page.

ISBN: 978-1-5043-9711-7 (sc)
ISBN: 978-1-5043-9713-1 (hc)
ISBN: 978-1-5043-9712-4 (e)

Library of Congress Control Number: 2018901549

Balboa Press rev. date: 03/15/2018

Contents

Heartfelt Acknowledgements

First and foremost, I'd like to extend my gratitude to my precious wife Ange and our three young children, for your love, your affection, your kindness, and your unreserved support in life and throughout the process of writing this book.

On a personal note, I extend my gratitude to my older brothers for being there for me as I was growing up without a father whom I lost at a young age. Thank you for your brotherly love and untiring strength.

I am grateful for the sweet and beautiful memories of my late father, mother and sisters, who all passed so early but left me with inspiring memories filled with love, grace, courage, hope and honor.

I extend my gratitude:

To Brother Rene D. Roy, a man who tirelessly and passionately kept opening doors of opportunity for a better education, not only for me but also for several dozen young people in need. I can never express the depth of my appreciation for your love, kindness, humility, and your unwavering support throughout these many years.

To Dr Paul Grand'Maison of the University of Sherbrooke for inspiring a whole generation of medical students through your love, affection, and through your warm presence which taught me more than words could ever hope to do. Thank you for your care and your support.

To Dr Beatrice Granger, Dr Guy Leveillé, Dr Stéphane Proulx, Dr Daniel St-Laurent, Dr Didier Jutras-Aswad, Dr Florence Chanut, Dr Cedric Andrès, Dr Michel Paradis, Dr Francine Morin, Dr Christiane Bertelli, Dr Amal Abdel Baki, Dr Rémi Coté, Dr Mimi Israel, Dr Serge Beaulieu, Dr Karine Goulet, Dr Pierre-Paul Yale, Dr Jacques Bernier, Dr. Mylène Valiquette-Lavigne, Dr Chantal Lemire, Dr Don Fujito, Dr Chris Abbott,

Dr Linda Jordan Platt and so many other mentors for your excellence in knowledge transmission, for your attention, for your support and for helping me shape my professional life.

To my former and present colleagues and collaborators from near and far, thank you for your presence, your fruitful discussions, and for your determination to make our world a better place.

I would like to thank my patients for helping me to grow not only professionally but also in my personal life. Your courage, your humility to ask for help, your perseverance and your determination to fight continues to inspire me every single day of my life.

To those of you who might be fighting the addiction of some kind, I commend your courage and personal conviction to fight for a better life.

I would like to acknowledge the efforts of those in the caring professions working tirelessly to help your patients rise above the burden of addiction. Whether you are a therapist, a doctor, a nurse, a rehab therapist, a family member, a spiritual or religious leader, or a community leader, I commend your courage and your tenacious spirit to help

Thank you to all of my friends, nieces, nephews and relatives, who help me stay balanced within this fast-paced and busy world; through your kindness, your love, your sense of humor, and the times we spend together, my life is richer and full of meaning. I extend my gratitude to my chosen family members Denis Auray and Fleurette Morin who played a great and love-filled parental role when I needed them most.

Finally, I'd like to extend my heartfelt gratitude to Thomas Layton-Smythe, Isabelle Carrière, Viviane Cholette, Jocelyne Bouchard, Eric Moses Gashirabake, Frédéric Ntawiniga for your professionalism and contributions throughout the process of editing, creating illustrations and for your resolved support in so many other ways throughout the process of publishing and sharing this book.

Introduction

"It's easy to stand with the crowd, it takes courage to stand alone."
—**Mahatma Gandhi**

I am writing this book out of love, out of passion, out of care for my fellow human beings, and out of personal duty. I feel the need to share and to engage my generation and the generations to come; I am writing to you because I believe in you! I believe in your ability to think and to cross-examine objective facts and most of all, I believe in your freedom and your capacity to learn and to make your own decisions based on your own process of investigating truth.

The idea to write this book birthed from the desire, the passion and personal mission to help inform the public about cannabis usage, and to bring about a much needed discussion about this drug with my fellow citizens of the world. As you have probably heard, several states in the United States of America and some countries in Europe have recently moved to legalize recreational marijuana usage, and Canada is in the process of legalizing the sale of recreational marijuana nation-wide. [1]

As I write, I can't help but imagine the fourteen, sixteen, or twenty-one-year-old young man or woman who might be wrestling with whether or not to try cannabis, but feel they don't have enough information to make an informed decision on one side of the argument or the other. I can't help but also consider the parents of this young person who might be wondering how to speak to their teenager about cannabis usage, or who may be struggling with whether or not to try the substance themselves.

Some people might argue that cannabis or marijuana is harmless and the proof is that it's being more and more legalized in different parts of the world, and others will argue that it's not because cannabis is being legalized that it's good for you, and they will say that tobacco smoking is legal but it remains very dangerous to your health.

This is not a book concerned with making judgements, it's not a book about telling you what to do or not to do, and it's not a book which wants to determine your choices for you; it's an informational tool using simple information and common language that anyone can understand. The intent of this book is to offer simple answers to commonly asked questions about cannabis...

What is cannabis? What changes can it make to your brain? Can it lead to mental health problems such as psychosis, depression, anxiety, or suicide? Can it lead to lung cancer? How might it affect your physical health? And what consequences might it have on your personal goals and ambitions, on your social relationships, and on your overall well-being? The goal of this book is not to judge anyone, but to provide you with illustrations, tables, basic scientific information, and easy to understand statistical tables about marijuana usage.

The purpose is to create awareness about this trivialized and supposedly harmless drug so that whatever choice we make at least we know we're making a well-advised and a well-educated choice to protect our brain, our young people's brains and to lovingly help free those who might already be oppressed by the burden of addiction.

We will mainly use the term *"cannabis"* in this book but we need to mention that *"marijuana"* is the term most commonly used around the world.

I will leave it up to you, the reader, to do the exercise of finding the *21 Unspoken Truths about Marijuana* as you progress through the reading. You may want to team up with a few other readers either directly or through a social media reading group to discuss your findings with them.

*There is a table found somewhere in the book that will help you examine whether you have explored all The 21 Unspoken Truths about Marijuana discussed in this book. That table contains all those twenty-one points.

Thank you for taking a few hours out of your precious time and hectic schedule to read and discuss the subject matter explored throughout this book, and I hope you are moved to share it with someone you care about!

Sincerely,

1

What is Cannabis?

"Drugs were a way of running from whatever it was I wanted to run from."
—Michael Phelps, winner of 28 Olympic medals.

Cannabis or Marijuana is the most commonly used illicit drug in the world and it is the most commonly used addictive substance after alcohol and tobacco. It is a natural plant which causes psychotropic effects on the brain when smoked or consumed and can cause real consequences in our everyday lives. Cannabis use is a topic worth discussing since it affects so many people and is present in so many homes. It affects not only individuals, but families, communities, as well as society as a whole. Multiple social, medical, political, and legislative issues are informed by cannabis usage; recreational marijuana, medical marijuana, treatment of addiction, and legislative factors are only a few of the societal issues that need to be considered by society at large. But let's not forget that cannabis use also affects individual lives as well; cannabis can be present in your life as a simple recreational or social issue, but it can also be an addiction issue, a financial issue, a family issue as it affects your relationships with family members, or a security issue as it affects your driving capabilities.

In this chapter, we will offer some simple information about this drug, we will discuss its history, slang terms, chemical components generally found in cannabis and basic statistics about the use of marijuana in the US, Canada, and throughout the world.

Stats Corner

- Cannabis, also known as marijuana, is the most commonly used addictive substance in the world after alcohol and tobacco [2-3-4]

- Most commonly used recreational drug in adolescents and young adults in the world [3-4]

- Within the US, 22.2 million people report that they have used cannabis within the past month according to the 2015 National Survey on Drug Use and Health

- Within Canada: usage is two to three times more frequent in youth (15-24) than in adults [5]

- **Increases in teenagers' emergency department visits related to cannabis have been observed in US states that have legalized recreational marijuana [6-7]**

- **Increases in marijuana use by teenagers and young adults have been observed in US states that have legalized recreational marijuana [6-7]**

Cannabis- What is it?

Cannabis, also known as marijuana, is a flowering plant.

Cannabis has been used as a drug for thousands of years.

Its use has been documented dating back to more than 2500 BC by Chinese emperors, Ancient Greeks and Romans

It's been used for recreational purposes, for medical purposes, and even for spiritual rituals in some societies.

There are three main species of cannabis: sativa, indica, and ruderalis, and these species are biologically very similar.

Sativa is the most commonly grown for recreational purposes.

Slang Terms for Cannabis

Marijuana, pot, cannabis, weed, wax, stone, hash, joint, herb, mj, reefer, dope, dob

There are more than 1,000 slang names [8]

How is Cannabis Consumed?

Can be smoked like a cigarette, called a marijuana joint

Can be rolled into a cigar, called a blunt

Can be smoked through a wide glass pipe, called a bong

Can be inhaled directly, through heating marijuana or hashish and inhaling the smoke

Can be ingested directly in marijuana teas, foods, candies, cookies, or other baked goods.

Cannabis: what gets you high?

Cannabis contains more than 500 different chemical compounds

Among these chemical components are compounds called cannabinoids

These cannabinoids bind to specific receptors in your brain called cannabinoid-receptors, and there are about one-hundred cannabinoids found in cannabis

The two main cannabinoids include: THC and Cannabidiol (CBD)

THC (tetrahydrocannabinol): This is the chemical compound responsible for getting you 'high' as well as causing other psychotropic effects.

Different THC concentrations of cannabis exist on the market.

And any cannabis with THC concentration above **10%** is considered **high** and potentially more harmful than cannabis with lower THC concentration.

A few decades ago Cannabis Potency or THC concentrations were much lower than they are today.

So if you feel that you absolutely have to use cannabis, at least check the concentrations of THC.

The more THC concentration in your cannabis, the more harmful to your mental health it might be.

Cannabidiol (CBD): This chemical has been mostly used for potential medical purposes.

Medical Marijuana

Marijuana has been used for medical purposes: it has been used in the treatment of epilepsy, chronic pain, increasing appetite and reducing nausea for chemotherapy patients. Research is ongoing for use in some immune system disorders and in military veterans living with symptoms of Post-Traumatic Stress Disorder.

But there is limited research in medical literature due mainly to the fact that it is difficult for researchers to get access to cannabis in conducting studies and medical trials.

Therefore, the majority of doctors do not prescribe cannabis to treat their patients in most countries.

2

What Happens When You Smoke, Inhale, Drink, or Eat Cannabis?

"We may encounter many defeats, but we must not be defeated"
—**Maya Angelou**

Cannabis is effective, it is fast, it has real effects on your body, your brain, your feelings and it certainly produces indisputably pleasurable effects; hence its appeal to people who choose to consume it. But consuming cannabis carries the risk of potential negative side effects, and may lead to serious consequences in some cases.

When you inhale cannabis…

When you smoke and inhale cannabis, the smoke travels to your lungs where it is absorbed into your bloodstream. It then circulates throughout your body and—most importantly—to your brain. Once there, it binds to cannabinoid receptors, stimulating the endocannabinoid system and the dopamine system in your brain. The circuitry responsible for addiction— also known as the dopamine reward system—is stimulated, causing sensations of pleasure. Cannabis also affects numerous other parts of your brain, producing a variety of reactions outlined in Table. 1- Cannabis in your brain in chapter 3. Smoking and inhaling cannabis produces rapid changes in the body and brain and its effects are felt almost immediately when consumed in this manner.

When you eat or drink cannabis…

When you eat or drink cannabis—for example, in a muffin, cake, or tea— the drug has to go through the digestive system before being absorbed into your bloodstream. Cannabis goes through the liver, where it is broken down or metabolized into other chemicals or metabolites. One chemical or metabolite produced in the liver is called 11-hydroxy-THC (11-OH-THC). This metabolite is even more potent or stronger than cannabis or THC itself. It can get you more mentally altered and its effects might last longer in your system. Therefore, when you eat or drink marijuana, the psychoactive effect takes longer to kick in—about thirty minutes or more—but the overall psychoactive effects can be increased with more loss of focus and balance, and more mental alteration than when marijuana is smoked or inhaled.

3

Cannabis in Your Brain

"Turn your wounds into wisdom."
—**Oprah Winfrey**

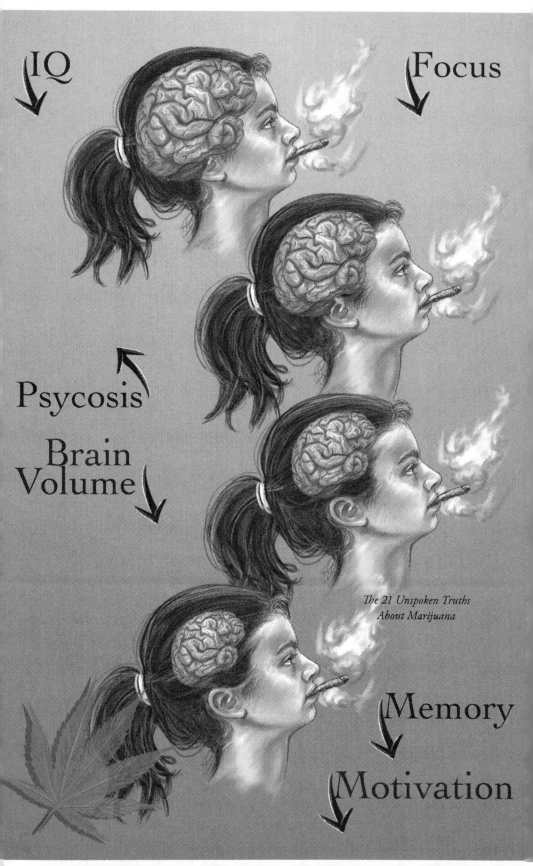

As we discussed throughout the previous chapter whether you smoke it, drink it, eat it, or inhale it, cannabis is absorbed into your blood which helps it travel to its favorite destination: your brain! Here it begins to act, either creating a 'buzz' (or a beautiful feeling), or 'getting you irrational'. It's in the delicate chemistry of the brain that marijuana acts to produce the desired—or undesirable—psychoactive effects, producing short and long-term consequences which are often hard to predict in advance.

Brain development is a very complex process; the brain starts to develop throughout the fetus' prenatal life and brain growth isn't entirely complete until around the age of twenty-five. So any physical, psychological or emotional trauma the brain experiences before the age of twenty-five is more likely to interfere with overall brain development, and is therefore more likely to cause long term damage to the brain.

Are you under 25 years old?

Cannabis has impacts on your brain at any age, but if you're under 25 years old, your brain is still developing and will be more affected by consuming it;

You are more at risk of developing an addiction to the drug, of developing symptoms of amotivational syndrome, learning problems, and even of developing a psychotic episode! These subjects will be discussed later in chapters 4, 7, 11, and 15.

Table 1 presents the different parts of the brain affected by cannabis consumption, as well as outlining some of the potential serious life consequences which could result from 'getting high'. However, it's important to acknowledge that this table is simplified, since the brain is complicated and its parts are more interconnected than can be fully outlined in any simple table! Any individual structure of the brain can be involved in controlling numerous aspects of how we behave; for example, the amygdala—one of the structures of the brain discussed in the table below—is involved both in our emotional reactions, as well as being involved in how we process memory, and in how we make decisions. Just remember that each part of the brain might also be affected by marijuana, and could subsequently affect other aspects of our behaviors not discussed below!

Table 1. How Cannabis/Marijuana Affects Your Brain

Structures of the Brain Affected by Cannabis	Function of Brain Structure	Effects of cannabis	Potential Life consequences
Hippocampus	Involved in memory...	↓memory	↑Learning problems
Orbitofrontal cortex	Involved in executive functions, focus, inhibition, judgement, planning...	↓judgement, ↓concentration, ↓attention span ↓behavioral inhibition ↓executive functions...	*↑Behavior problems, *↑impulsivity *↓judgment *↑sexual behavior with no attachment *↑risk of addiction *↑Risk of accidents, *↓ability to learn...
Cerebellum	Involved in balance, movement, coordination...	Reduced balance and coordination...	*↑Risk of fall, *↑Risk of accidents
Basal ganglia	Involved in movement planning and Coordination...	*slower in reacting to sudden events *↓movement planning and coordination	↑risk of car accidents
Amygdala	Involved in fear and aggressive behavior, anxiety, emotions...	If high doses of cannabis: ↑Fear ↑Anxiety ↑panic...	*Anxiety problems *panic *isolation *aggressiveness *depressive mood...
Hypothalamus	Involved in hormonal control, appetite, sleep, attachment behavior...	↑appetite and eating, ↑sleep dysregulation, ↓attachment.	*↑appetite and eating *long term sleep problems, *↑sexual behavior with no attachment, *↓attachment to one's family...
Overall brain anatomy	-↓brain volume -thinning of the cerebral cortex -changes in cerebral white matter -in addition to the functional changes noted above [26]		

4

Cannabis: Teenagers, Young Adults

"Courage is what it takes to stand up and talk, courage is also what it takes to sit down and listen."
—**Winston Churchill**

Psychosis

Cannabis increases the risk of psychosis

By 40% for occasional users;

By 390% for heavy and regular users;

Brain continues to develop up until age of 25 years

Stay away, especially if you're under 25 years' old

Intelligence

↓ IQ
↓ Focus
↓ Attention span
↓ Memory,

↑Car Accidents

Amotivational Syndrome

↑ School failure
↑ Unemployment
↓ Motivation
↓ Ambition

Lung Cancer

deterioration of respiratory diseases

-In our mother's womb, during the third week of fetus development, our brain begins to form...

- This process of brain development continues until around the age of twenty-five.[9,26]

-Therefore, it is extremely important to be careful with what substances the brain is exposed to during this vulnerable period, since changes to the partially developed brain can last a lifetime!

As life begins, so does the formation of the brain. Your brain starts developing in your mother's womb. At the very beginning of the fetus' third week, cells begin to clump together to begin creating what will arguably become the most crucial organ in your body, the pilot of your life, the host of your mind, the chief controller and the maestro of your organs: your brain!

This process includes the growth of different brain structures as well as the formation of crucial connections which link different parts of the brain together. It also involves the trimming of unnecessary connections over time, a process known as 'synaptic pruning'.

Your brain continues to develop and mature over the next twenty-five years. The final parts of the brain to develop are the frontal lobes; these parts are mainly involved in planning, anticipating future events, paying attention and focusing, decision making, inhibitory control, reasoning, and problem solving.

Imagine for a moment what might happen to your brain if it is exposed to a toxic substance, or to a physical or emotional trauma while it is still in the process of developing; this might slow or interfere with brain development in different ways, and might have future impacts which could be hard to predict!

> **So your thirteen-year-old or fifteen-year-old brain, or even your twenty-one-year-old brain is—unfortunately—much more vulnerable to being altered by cannabis than a forty-year-old brain would be.**

As we discuss in chapter three and chapter nine, cannabis, especially when repetitively used by teenagers, might lead to cognitive dysfunction, difficulty controlling impulsive behaviors, reduced capacity in problem solving, reduced focus and attention and temporary drop in IQ among many other negative effects discussed in those chapters. Let us underline that these negative effects might not be fully reversible.

Also, as will be discussed in later chapters, adolescents and young adults who try cannabis are at increased risk of developing an addiction to cannabis sometime within their adult life, and are also at much higher risk of experiencing a psychotic episode as compared to adults who try marijuana.....

Stats Corner

> **1 in 9 cannabis users will become dependent** [10,11,12]
>
> - **These risks almost double for adolescents**
>
> - **About 17% of adolescents who try or use cannabis will become dependent**
>
> - **That's about 1 in 6 adolescents who will become dependent to cannabis if they try it!**
>
> - **The risk of addiction to cannabis increases between 25 to 50 % for those who use it daily.**

5

Cannabis: Pregnancy and Breastfeeding

"Do what you can, with what you have, where you are."
—Theodore Roosevelt

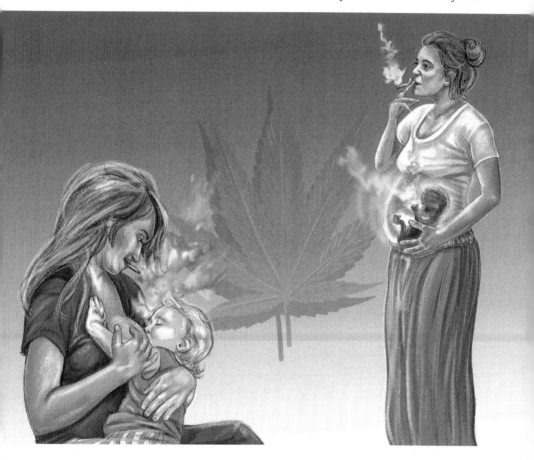

---

*When a mother smokes, the fetus smokes, the baby smokes

-Cannabis—specifically THC and its other cannabinoids—cross the placental barrier, so the fetus is exposed if the mother smokes, drinks, or eats cannabis products.[13]

- The breastfed baby is also exposed to cannabis through the milk if the mother is smoking, drinking or eating cannabis products.

-Cannabis second hand smoke, just like in tobacco, is also to be avoided.

Cannabis, and especially THC, is known to cross the placental barrier, and about ten to thirty percent of the cannabis circulating in the mother's blood will cross into the fetus' system. Cannabis is also present in the mother's milk, so the breastfed baby may also be exposed to the drug if the mother is a marijuana user.

More research is needed to study the long term effects of using cannabis during pregnancy, but some studies have suggested that it might have lasting effects on the child's behavior throughout childhood and adolescence. Children and teenagers who were exposed to cannabis during their gestation might be more impulsive, more irritable, have difficulty with focus, attention, problem solving, anticipation and planning.[14,15,16]

6

Who Becomes Addicted and who Does Not?

"Tis one thing to be tempted, another thing to fall."
—William Shakespeare

> **When we submit to the temptation of achieving pleasure and instant gratification, it comes at a personal cost.**
>
> **When we find ourselves compromising our morals, our principles, our careers, our future goals, our families' well-being, and our health to achieve that "feel good" moment—and find ourselves doing so over and over again—here we can start talking about addiction.**

Can anyone become addicted to cannabis? Who is more at risk of succumbing to cannabis addiction? Can some people use cannabis without becoming addicted?

As you probably already know, it's in human beings' nature and design to seek out what's most pleasurable, enjoyable, and least difficult; it is only when we are following a greater purpose to achieve our goals that we choose to take a more difficult path. We all long for pleasure and the faster and easier we can obtain it, the more we risk becoming addicted to the source of pleasure. The design of the human mind allows us to experience enjoyment, but also makes us vulnerable to becoming addicted to these pleasurable experiences…

How do we biologically fall into addiction?

The Reward System or Dopamine reward pathways

Our brain is intelligently designed; the circuitry of our brain is designed to help us enjoy pleasurable activities such as great meals, good company with friends, or a stimulating encounter with a new romantic interest. The brain circuitry system responsible for allowing us to enjoy such experiences is called the Reward System or the dopamine reward pathways. These pathways in the brain encourage us to seek out these awesome, exciting, and pleasurable experiences and reinforces these types of behaviors when we seek them out, making us more likely to do so over time. Let us underscore that there are survival reasons to this reward system, food is pleasurable to encourage us to eat and stay alive, sex is pleasurable to encourage us to mate and reproduce.

You can skip the following paragraph if you're not interested in scientific explanations, but if you are, let's briefly discuss the structures of your brain which are involved in developing addictive behaviors. The reward system is first stimulated when an addictive substance or pleasurable experience is encountered; practically all addictive substances will directly or indirectly increase dopamine levels in your brain. Dopamine is a neurotransmitter or chemical in your brain that is involved in pleasure and motivation. Without going into detailed medical or scientific explanations of this circuitry, let us note that the reward system involves many parts of the brain such as the prefrontal cortex, the nucleus accumbens, the limbic system, the anterior cingulate, the ventral tegmental area, and the amygdala…

When exposed to an addictive substance, the reward circuitry stimulates some people to seek more intense experiences to achieve the same pleasure over time. As someone repetitively uses the drug, dopamine is released and over time the brain becomes 'used to' the dopamine released by the brain, it then releases less dopamine for the same amount of stimulation-or same amount of substance-over time, and therefore requires ever larger amounts of stimulation to achieve the same pleasure as time progresses. Furthermore, the brain's response is dependent on numerous other factors such as genetic predisposition, morals, self-control, life stressors, protective factors, etc., and so everyone's vulnerability to addiction is based on a variety of different variables.

In these cases, the need to achieve pleasure becomes an affliction; feeling good becomes the ultimate goal, and the person can become trapped by compulsive instant gratification seeking behavior.

When we submit to the temptation of achieving pleasure and instant gratification, it comes at a personal cost.

> **When we find ourselves compromising our morals, our principles, our careers, our future goals, our families' well-being, and our health to achieve that "feel good" moment—and find ourselves doing so over and over again—here we can start seeing the signs of addiction.**

Our Brains might look similar, but each Brain is Unique!

All brains are based on a shared basic design, but they are not identical. We see variations in sizes of different brains, in the sizes of different structures of the brain, variations in the connections between different parts of the brain, and functional differences which neuroscientists can't yet fully explain or understand. Some brains are more vulnerable to addiction or mental health problems than others, for a variety of reasons. Two people from the same background, at the same age, and in comparable health could ingest the same drug, and while one will be fine, the other could experience a psychotic episode! We are all unique, and due to a host of genetic, emotional, and nurturing differences, we might all be affected in unique ways if we choose to use drugs.

Who gets Addicted and Who does not?

Stats Corner

> - **Not all drugs or alcohol users become addicted**
>
> - **About 10% to 20% of all substance users will lose control and slide into addiction** [17]
>
> - **50% of the risk of substance addiction can be attributed to genetic factors** [17]
>
> - **Additional risk factors are involved in triggering the addiction, if the user is exposed to addictive substances.**
>
> - **Teenagers and Young Adults are at higher risk of becoming addicted to cannabis**

So the question is: can anyone become addicted to cannabis or other drugs? The tricky answer is both "yes" and "no". Given the right circumstances, the right substances, the right experiences, and the right timing, I believe anyone can develop an addiction of some kind. Some might become addicted to cannabis, others to cocaine, alcohol, or amphetamines. Others still to pornography, internet usage, cellphones or social media, videogames, or to watching sports. Those who are vulnerable, like the high sensation seekers or novelty-seekers, are at increased risk whenever they engage in thrill-seeking or pleasure-seeking behaviors which expose them to the possibility of becoming addicted.

Some studies suggest that about 10% to 20% percent of substance users will become addicted to the substances they consume.[17] Genetics plays a major role in determining who will or won't become addicted to substances, and researchers suggest up to 50% of this risk is determined by your genetic predisposition to addictive behaviors in the first place.[17] Many other risk factors also play a role, such as life stressors, family history, brain developmental stage and age, and the type of drugs being consumed. Teenagers are far more vulnerable to developing an addiction when they try an addictive substance than adults are.

7

Addiction Risk Factors

"There are only two ways to live your life. One is as though nothing is a miracle. The other is as though everything is a miracle."

—Albert Einstein

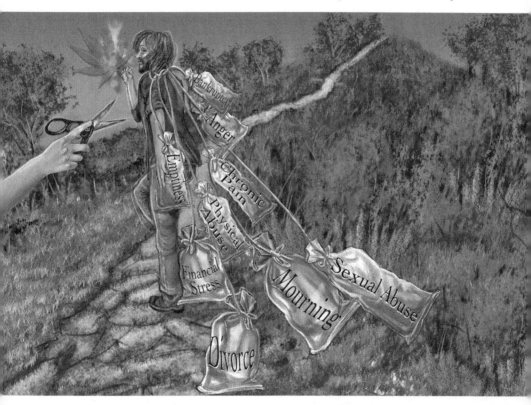

Table 2.

Do you have a parent, sibling, or relative who has struggled with a drug or alcohol addiction?
Are you addicted to alcohol or other substances right now, or do you feel you've shown addictive behaviors in the past?
Are you going through a tough time in your life?
Do you feel emotionally fragile or vulnerable at this moment?
Are you hanging around people who are using cannabis or other drugs, or do you have easy access to drugs?
Are you suffering from anxiety or depression?
Are your parents going through a separation or divorce?
Are you going through a break up or divorce yourself?
Do you feel you've had a traumatic childhood?
Have you experienced physical, sexual, or psychological abuse in the past?
Are you under financial stress, or having a difficult time making ends meet?
Are you experiencing conflicts at home?
Would you describe your family as being dysfunctional?
Are you a teenager or young adult?
Do you have a diagnosis of Attention Deficit and Hyperactivity Disorder (ADHD), or suspect that you might have the condition?
Are you suffering from a personality disorder?
Are you suffering from a psychotic disorder?
Do you often gamble, or find it hard to stop gambling when you start in the first place?
Have you recently lost your job, or have you been experiencing stress and conflict in the workplace?

If you said "yes" to any of the questions above, you may be at increased risk of abusive or addictive usage of cannabis, alcohol, or other drugs. But even if you answered "no" to all of these questions, this doesn't completely eliminate your risk, since it's difficult to predict how any individual might react to taking drugs for the first time!

One way or the other, these questions highlight some of the major risk factors which distinguish "social" users of cannabis from those who tend to fall into drug abuse and dependence. Having one or more of these risk factors does not imply that you are doomed to develop an addiction, it simply means that the statistical risk is increased. For example, if your father had a drug addiction problem, it's statistically more likely that you would develop a drug problem as well, but it does not necessarily mean that you are condemned to that problem yourself!

Family History: A Big Risk Factor!

- **We have zero control on the family we are born into, we do not chose our genetic makeup, or our biology.**

- **We not only inherit our genes from our family, but we also learn our habits, our understanding of life, and of the ways to cope with challenges and obstacles we face.**

- **But, we are not condemned to live our lives like they did!**

As stated previously, fifty percent of the risk of developing an addiction can be attributed to your genetic background. But fortunately, we are made up of more than just our genes! Generally, additional risk factors also play a role; it takes cumulative biological, environmental, and psychosocial factors to trigger an addiction.

In addition to genetic predisposition to addictive behaviors, we also have a tendency to repeat what we know, what we see, and what's been around us during our formative years. If you grow up with abusive drug use in your environment, you're more likely to re-enact the same behaviors.

The tough reality is that we cannot choose our family, we cannot decide where we are born or where we grow up. We aren't free to choose our family background. This means we face a bigger mountain to climb, a bigger challenge to overcome when raised within a dysfunctional family or a family marred by substance abuse. If this is your situation, you may wish to avoid addictive substances altogether since you face a greater risk of becoming addicted should you choose to try them. If you have a family history of alcohol or drug abuse—meaning a parent, brother, sister, cousin, uncle or aunt, or grandparent abused these substances—I suggest you avoid addictive substances such as cannabis because of the increased risk of developing an addiction yourself.

> There is a bigger mountain to climb, a bigger challenge to overcome, a larger wave to surf when you come from a dysfunctional family or a family marred by substance abuse. But you can still overcome.

Trauma in your Past?

If you've gone through traumatic life experiences in your past such as verbal, physical, or sexual abuse, your ability to regulate your emotions might be weakened, your stress coping mechanisms might be shaky, the ability to cope with stress is fragile, the real trust in people might be broken, your choices might be compromised, the fear can be deafening and the self-confidence might be sleeping. If you combine this psychological risk factors with social, biological and environmental risk factors, the risk of falling into addiction might be greatly increased....Be aware, and take care!

Life Stressors

During stressful life circumstances, a stress hormone called cortisol-increases in your brain and body, It might be tempting to consider using drugs such as cannabis to provide temporary relief and "feel good" moments during particularly challenging times. However, the temporary relief drugs might bring us can easily become a sensation we begin to miss and return to experience over and over again. By seeking respite from stressful life events, we might unwittingly find ourselves slipping into drug abuse.

It's important to note that not all those who try drugs will become addicted; only ten to twenty percent of drugs users will lose control and fall into drug abuse or dependence. Science still can't fully explain why some people remain in control of their drug use, but we know that biogenetic factors, psychological factors, social and environmental stressors, life development stage, and family history all play a role.[17]

Table 3: Biological, Psychosocial, and Environmental Risk Factors for Developing a Drug Dependence

Biological Risk Factors	- Genetic Predisposition
	- Stage of development of your brain (ex. adolescent, young adult)
	- Medical condition (ex. Chronic pain...)
	- Psychiatric conditions (Depression, anxiety, psychotic disorders, schizophrenia, bipolar disorder, personality disorders, ADHD...)
	- Abuse of other substances
Risk Factors related to a history of Trauma	- Physical abuse victim
	- Sexual abuse victim
	- Psychological abuse victim
	- Bullying victim

Social-Environmental Risk Factors	- Experiencing divorce, separation, relationship break-up, or being the child of parents going through a divorce or separation
	- Experiencing Peer pressure
	- Experiencing Economic stress
	- Experiencing Stressful life Events (ex. New job, new relationship, wedding),….
	- Friend group or close relatives who use drugs
	- Easy access to the drug
	- Judicial or Employment problems
	- Chaotic home Life
	- Grieving the Loss of a loved one…
	- Growing up with a feeling of rejection
	- Growing up fatherless or motherless

8

How Do You Know You're Sliding from Cannabis Use Into Abuse?

"You may have to fight a battle more than once, to win it."
—**Margaret Thatcher**

Stats Corner

- 1 in 9 marijuana users will slide into addiction

- These risks almost double for teenagers

- about 17% or 1 in 6 teenagers who try cannabis will show signs of addiction.[10,11,12]

*The risk of dependence might jump to 25-50% for those who use marijuana on daily basis.

Quick reflection Questions

Are you consuming more cannabis than you originally intended to?

Are you consuming cannabis more frequently?

Are you hiding your drug use from your loved ones?

Are you having conflicts with your family or friends about your drug use?

Are you lying about your substance use?

Are you having financial problems because of your drug use?

Are you neglecting your responsibilities due to your drug use?

Are you neglecting family relationships or close friends?

Are you prioritizing peers who share your habit and neglecting other meaningful social interactions?

If you answered "yes" to any of the above questions, you may be at increased risk of abusing cannabis—or have potentially already fallen into that category! Many people who are becoming addicted or are regularly abusing drugs might still be in denial about their actions; you may not share others' views about the dangers and risks associated with your own drug consumption or your behaviors when using drugs. Do you ever find yourself getting into heated discussions or conflicts with loved ones, or accuse them of exaggerating when it comes to the frequency of your drug use?

When you start receiving criticism from the people close to you about your use of addictive substances, when you start experiencing guilt or shame, when you find yourself unable to control the quantity you consume or when you start taking more than you intended to, when you're tempted to lie to your friends or family about your substance use, when you experience withdrawal symptoms on those occasions when you choose to refrain, when you start to ignore meaningful social interactions because you're either focused on finding the drug or hanging out with peers who share your habit, when you start to ignore your usual responsibilities or activities or start needing the drug to be able to sleep or relax, then you know you are probably sinking into marijuana abuse or addiction.

9

A Gateway Drug-A Front Door Drug

Can Marijuana Use Lead to The Abuse of Other Drugs?

"A journey of a thousand miles begins with a single step."
—**Lao Tzu**

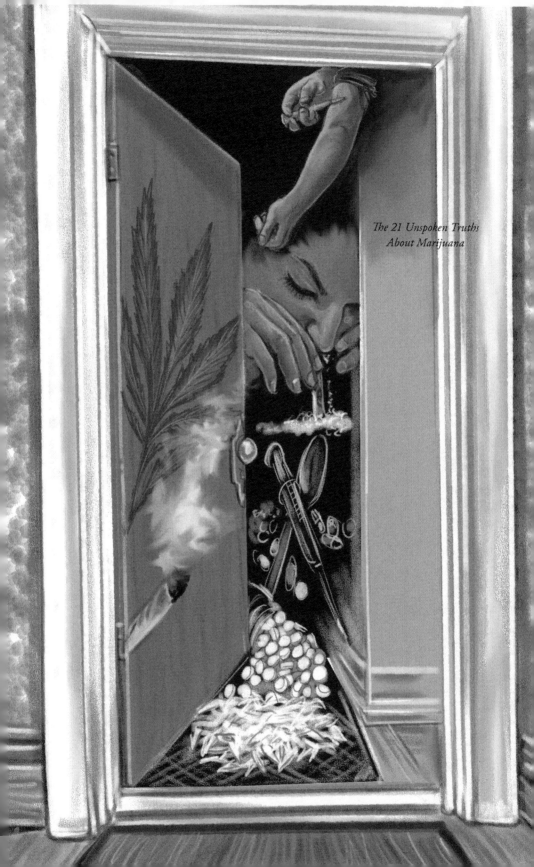

The 21 Unspoken Truths About Marijuana

Marijuana, a gateway drug? A Front Door drug?

-If you use marijuana, especially during adolescent years or as a young adult, you have an increased risk of developing addictions to other illicit drugs later in life.[18,19,20,21]

-It's also true for other drugs, including alcohol and tobacco, the addiction to any substance is associated with a higher risk of falling into addiction to other substances or illicit drugs.[18,19,20,21]

The use of cannabis during vulnerable stages of brain development can lead to changes to your endocannabinoid system, and consequently cause permanent changes to your dopamine reward pathway. Additionally, it could interfere with the maturing process of other crucial parts of the brain involved in behavior inhibition and decision, such as the prefrontal cortex. These brain chemistry changes contribute to increasing the risks for teenagers and young adults who are exposed to cannabis to seeking more powerful psychoactive drugs throughout their lifetime.

While the majority of cannabis users might not abuse other drugs later on, researchers have noticed that those who use cannabis as teenagers are at higher statistical risk of developing drug dependency behaviors with other illicit drugs later in life; [18,19,20,21] this tendency is what some people are referring to when they call cannabis "a gateway drug". It's important however to clarify that this tendency is also true of all other drugs, not just marijuana; the abuse of any substance—including alcohol and tobacco—is associated with increased risks of developing other substance addictions.

10

Can Cannabis Lead To Intellectual Decline or Cognitive Dysfunction?

"There are those that look at things the way they are, and ask why? I dream of things that never were, and ask why not?"
—**Robert F. Kennedy**

As discussed in chapter 3, marijuana affects different parts of your brain; memory is temporarily affected and chronic use can even affect the hippocampus, which is one of the main structures of the brain involved in memory retention. Cannabis also affects the prefrontal cortex, involved in behavior inhibition, focus, attention, planning, organization and anticipation; potential long term effects on these brain areas associated with chronic marijuana usage can lead to learning problems, academic or even professional failures. In fact, regular cannabis users can see their I.Q score drop almost 10 points! We need to note that cognitive effects of marijuana might not be fully reversible once marijuana consumption ceases.

Stat corner:

-For some heavy and regular adolescent cannabis users ° I.Q score might drop almost 10 points, [22]

-This might not be reversible even when they stop consuming cannabis during adulthood.[22]

11

Amotivational Syndrome: can cannabis kill my career, my ambitions, & my dreams?

"Courage is like a muscle; it is strengthened by use"
—**Ruth Gordon**

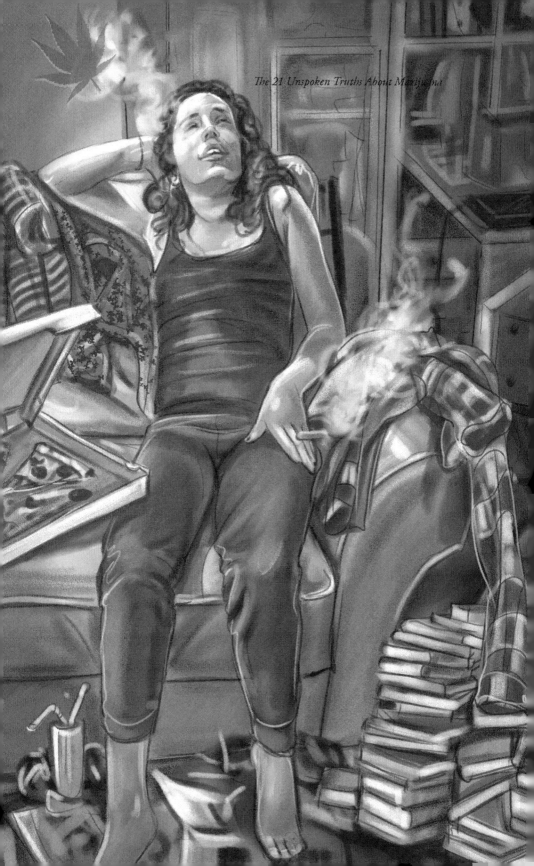

> **For many cannabis and substance abusers the motivation towards pleasure-seeking and instant gratification sometimes overtakes the real motivation towards a more ambitious, fulfilling, balanced and goal-oriented life.**
>
> **When addiction takes over, soon the "high life" replaces the real life! The feck life becomes the life.**

Picture an eighteen-year-old student, a great guy with a positive attitude who is highly motivated, ambitious, and intelligent. This student is both academically and socially active, is close to his mother, and is very helpful in pitching in around the house with any necessary domestic chores.

Little by little, this portrait of him starts to change; he begins getting into more frequent conflicts with his mom, loses interest towards getting good grades, spends less time with his family and increasing amounts of time outside the home. He no longer wants to set challenging goals for himself anymore, and all his ambitious life-plans start to go downhill. He makes new friends—mainly toxic friends, whom his mother disapproves of—and his childhood best friends are shown the door, one by one.

His ultimate goal becomes instant gratification; he spends his time listening to music, smoking "weed", chilling with friends, and telling each other stories in noisy smoke-filled apartments and bars. Our student's need for pleasure overtakes his motivation to live a more fulfilling, balanced, ambitious, and goal-oriented life. The "high life" replaces real life…

> **This lifestyle of drug use associated with a shift in personal goals, this lethargy, this loss of motivation, this lack of ambition and purpose, this neglect of priorities, this apathy is what is commonly described by health professionals as "Amotivational Syndrome".**

This syndrome is one of the most common side effects associated with chronic cannabis usage, one which is shared with almost all other addictions as well. When taken regularly, cannabis has serious impacts on your level of motivation and often traps users in a cycle of lethargy and apathy which can last for months or years at a time, without accessing the proper help.

Cannabis can absolutely distract you from thinking about your ambitions, and leave your dreams by the wayside. Chronic marijuana consumption creates its own selfish meaning in your life; it starts scheduling regular appointments with you on a daily basis, and soon you start looking forward to that beautiful relaxation time you are spending with your weed every day at the expense of everything else you used to find important.

Smoking a joint or "vaping weed" becomes the best moment of your day, and spending time thinking about your goals, ambitions, and dreams becomes optional. Spending time with your marijuana-using friends rises to the top of your priority list, while spending time with your family and caring friends falls to the bottom of the list. Real friends, real family, real goals, and real dreams suddenly are perceived to be boring. Making jokes with fake and superficial friends while smoking marijuana takes precedence over all else, while the people who care about you the most begin to increasingly worry about your well-being.

> **Over the longer term, amotivational syndrome often leads to a dysfunctional and deficient lifestyle. Professional, academic, and social failures keep piling up, feelings of self-worth and confidence decrease, and depression starts knocking on our door.**

While the symptoms of amotivational syndrome are often mistaken for those of depression, they are both separate mental health conditions. However, the consequences of losing one's interest in previously loved activities and ceasing to engage in meaningful social interactions and relationships often leads to symptoms of depression over the longer term. So it's worth knowing how to detect amotivational syndrome if you begin to recognize its negative consequences in your own behavior, since they can sometimes lead us down a path of lifestyle choices which might be impossible to reverse.

12

Cannabis: Social Life and Family Relationships

"When wealth is lost, nothing is lost. When health is lost, something is lost. When character is lost, everything is lost."
—**Billy Graham**

> **When overwhelmed by drug addiction, sadly**
>
> - **what's easy becomes the goal, what's immediate becomes the focus, what's feck becomes cool, the quick pleasure becomes the aim, immediate gratification becomes the purpose.**
> - **What's lasting becomes optional, what's hard becomes annoying, what's real becomes uncool, what's worthy becomes tasteless and what's long becomes pointless.**

Can cannabis negatively affect your relationships?

Before going any further in this discussion, it will be useful to keep in mind that there is a difference between a social life based on obtaining pleasure versus one which is based on principals and achieving fulfillment.

You can socialize often, be surrounded constantly by others, yet still feel lonely; you can have numerous people in your life, yet still feel isolated!

This may seem like a contradictory statement, but it speaks to a truth which I observe every day in my profession as a psychiatrist. There are people who spend their teenage years, their twenties, or even their middle age wasting so much of their valuable time nurturing superficial relationships focused around achieving pleasure and simple gratification. These individuals surround themselves with many frivolous friends, and involve themselves in numerous activities, yet forgot to nurture long-lasting relationships that truly matter. They focus so intently on pleasurable activities that they forget the true meaning of happiness, which is the attainment of a well-balanced life.

> **We can socialize a lot, be with people a lot, be surrounded a lot, yet still feel lonely. We can have numerous people in our life, yet still feel isolated.**

Getting back to the subject of marijuana, using the drug can certainly provide relief for some people, may cause physically pleasurable sensations (and potentially lead to the occasional laughing fit), but it would be difficult to say that it necessarily leads to a permanent state of fulfillment or happiness. The pleasurable feelings associated with marijuana can be very sneaky, since when ingesting marijuana becomes a person's ultimate goal the person will sometimes end up resorting to deceptive behavior to maintain their habit, like lying to the family or partner, misusing family finances, sometimes stealing, neglecting family and personal priorities and so forth. This priority shift was discussed in the chapter on amotivational syndrome.

Some people argue that cannabis has the capacity to increase social interactions with friends but neglect to mention the type and quality of increased social interactions; yes, it may increase pleasure of being within a social group, the desire to spend more time with peers who share the same habits, but it may also distance you from those friends who disagree with your drug consumption behavior, and potentially isolate you from those who attempt to get you back on the road towards achieving your dreams.

> - **Cannabis usage, especially when it veers towards addiction, may decrease the pleasure you feel spending sober time with your family, and with your ambitious and goal oriented friends.**
>
> - **It may increase your desire for pleasurable, yet superficial, impermanent social interactions, and decrease your interest in nurturing long lasting social ties based in sobriety.**
>
> - **These social tendencies are observed in the social relationships of almost all addicts!**

13

Peer Pressure

"When you say 'Yes' to others, make sure you are not saying 'No' to yourself."
—**Paolo Coelho**

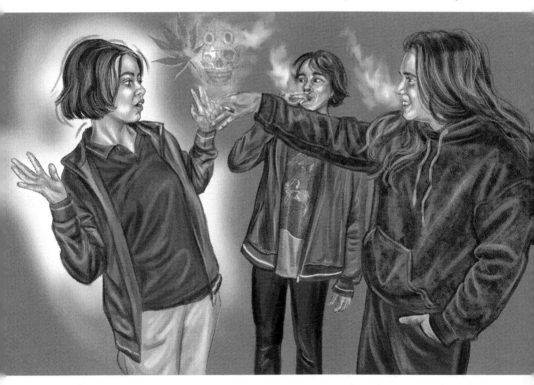

Stats Corner

> - **Cannabis is the most commonly used addictive drug after tobacco and alcohol** [24]
>
> - **The rate of adolescents' and young adults'(15-24) cannabis usage is 2 times higher than that of adults 25 years and older** [5]
>
> - **22.5 million Americans have used cannabis within the previous month based on a 2015 national survey** [2]

While it's comforting to feel we belong somewhere, and it's clear that loneliness, rejection, solitude, and difficulty making friends are painful experiences, the neediness and desperation with which we seek feelings of acceptance and love can sometimes lead us to accept very high personal costs.

Consider the case of a certain fourteen-year-old girl, rejected and abandoned by her dad, psychologically abused by her mother, and sexually abused by numerous of her mother's boyfriends. Feelings of loneliness are practically inscribed on an invisible sign hanging around her neck! Without friends, she's been moving more than twice a year with her mother for many years; she has been rejected and bullied so badly, that she's been forced to switch schools four times since having started secondary school two years ago. She feels alone at home and at school, and desperately needs to be accepted at all costs.

She is invited by a cool group of older schoolmates to join their table, and she feels accepted and taken care of; for the first time since having started high school, she no longer feels afraid of being bullied, and she begins to spend as much time as possible with her new friends, much of which is spent smoking marijuana. Her new gang becomes a part of her everyday life and she has a lot of fun, but it's not all positive; she also experiences a lot of hurt along the way. She begins to realize that her acceptance in the group is conditional on continuing to behave like the group, talk like the group, share the same lifestyle as the group, and dress like her friends. In becoming like the group, she is not free to totally be herself. She cannot make her own decisions, dress as she wishes, or think for herself; she finds the group's acceptance and affection is entirely conditional on behaving as they wish.

Compromising her basic principles becomes her new norm; the more she compromises, the more she smokes marijuana, the more her judgement is affected, and the more lost she becomes. Depression sets in, and she begins to set fewer goals for herself, and the more suicidal she becomes as the years pass.

Submitting to peer pressure to seek acceptance, affection, or because of fear comes with a very big price. The big question you should ask yourself: is it worth the cost? Surrendering to peer pressure might cost you your positive relationships with your family members, your real friends, your financial savings, and your health or ultimately even your life!

When all is said and done it's okay to accept risks in life, but before you make the decision to make using drugs a part of your life, ask yourself again: am I more vulnerable? Am I at higher risk of addiction or psychosis? If so, is it worth the risk? Once you've done this, go ahead and decide what's best for you knowing that you've looked at the situation clearly.

- Is it worth risking developing an addiction, is it worth risking your family, your real friends, is it worth risking psychosis, depression, or even suicide just to be accepted, just to fit in, just to please those friends who will not be around a few years from now? Is it worth the possible price?

- If you're an adolescent you're at increased risk of surrendering to peer pressure and you are more suggestible than the adults are

If you use Cannabis, especially during adolescent years or as a young adult, you have an increased risk of developing addictions to other illicit drugs later in life.[18,19,20,21]

14

Can using Cannabis lead to symptoms of Depression and Anxiety?

"Try to be a rainbow in someone's cloud"
—**Maya Angelou**

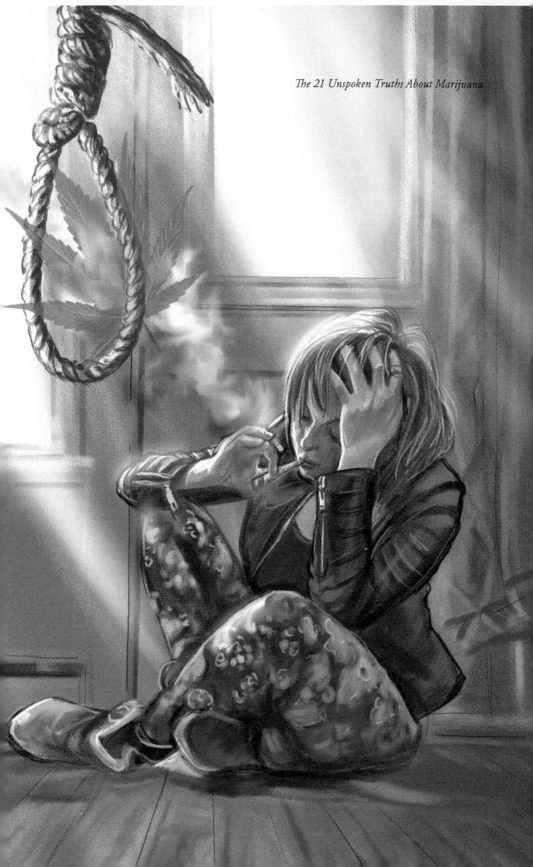

> **Marijuana can make you feel good in the moment, but that longed for 'feel-good moment' can play tricks on us;**
>
> **When use turns to abuse, marijuana could be a 'smoke-screen' hiding our profound suffering and pain, symptoms that will only become obvious to us later on down the road of life.**

One of the reasons marijuana is popular and is so commonly used by adolescents and by young adults is that it makes some people feel good, in fact, very good. It can certainly decrease anxiety for some time, and some even use it on a daily basis before going to bed, as they feel they can't sleep without its beautiful powers of relaxation. But is there anything else hidden behind that beautiful feeling? Is it a great gift from nature, or could it be a rose with thorns?

Neglecting the Cornerstones

When we fall into an addiction of any kind, there is a tendency to neglect certain aspects of our lives, and sometimes crucial cornerstones are carelessly set aside. But we can be all-but-certain that those ignored pieces will be missing later on down the line when we will be needing them the most!

We can choose to seek immediate gratification through marijuana, we can enjoy superficial relief from our problems and negative feelings, we can hang out with superficial people and ignore major pieces of the puzzle like family, work, physical exercise, and significant relationships. But when we are finally reminded of what we've been missing—as we fall back to the reality of solid ground—we are eventually forced to confront the consequences which accompany the easy choices and quick fixes we chose to make earlier on.

When you realize that you've been living in a static way—enjoying the moment, but not advancing anywhere, while everyone else has kept progressing—regrets begin to arise and you may start to blame either your own behavior, circumstances beyond your control, or the people who surround you. Anxiety starts settling in, as do worries, and regrets about missed past opportunities. When we realize we have few realistic prospects for future opportunities, depression starts knocking at the door, and then it enters and makes itself at home!

> **You take drugs to try to diffuse the emotional pain, but the more you take, the more anxious you become. The more anxious you become, the more you take to try to ease the pain, yet become even less functional and experience even more emotional pain.**
>
> **You return to marijuana again and again for the 'buzz' you need to freeze this pain, but only end up leading yourself down the path of an ever deepening cycle filled with amotivational syndrome, professional failures, regrets, and symptoms of depression.**

Additionally, it's important to remember that cannabis affects many parts of your brain simultaneously, including the amygdala which is the part of the brain involved in the regulation of our emotions. When you consume large quantities of cannabis, the amygdala is affected and you may subsequently experience symptoms of fear or anxiety, or even panic attacks. If you have a family history of depression or anxiety, feel you are suffering from a drug or alcohol addiction, if you are a teenager or young adult under the age of twenty-five, if you're experiencing stressful life events which could increase your risk of becoming addicted, you may wish to avoid using marijuana altogether—at least for now—since the risks could be far greater than any relief or pleasure you might reasonably hope to experience from using the drug.

> **Cannabis literarily affects the parts of your brain, like amygdala, that regulate anxiety, fear and emotions. When you take high quantities of cannabis, the areas involved in emotional and fear regulation are affected and then you can see your anxiety skyrocketing and for some people it can even result in panic attacks and depression.**

15

Can cannabis lead to psychosis or schizophrenia?

"I learned that courage was not the absence of fear, but the triumph over it. The brave man is not who that does not feel afraid but he who conquers that fear."
—**Nelson Mandela**

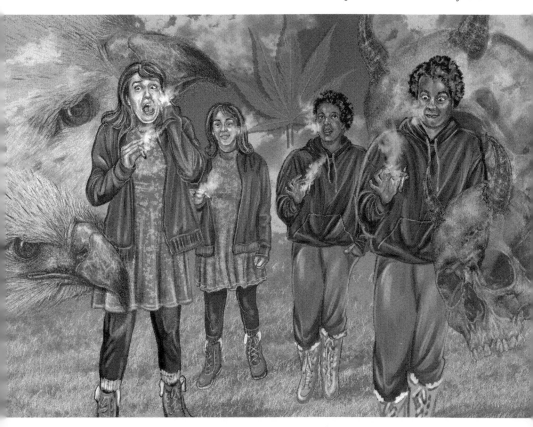

Can I take cannabis if I am a teenager?

Can I take cannabis if I am under 25 years old?

The answer to these questions is: not without a potentially big risk!

Can using cannabis lead to a psychotic episode or onset of schizophrenia?

Young lives can indeed sometimes be cut short by marijuana abuse, as this story illustrates: at the time of his death he was thirty years old, an aspiring song writer, and a great guy who is still missed by his friends to this day. From the first time he smoked pot, he experienced symptoms of psychosis as he repeatedly lost contact with reality, and believed himself to have super powers and was paranoid with feeling of persecution. These psychotic episodes could last between a few hours to a few weeks, but during his last time using marijuana, he took such a large amount of the drug that his judgement was completely distorted, and believing himself to be invincible and immortal, the man jumped from a dangerous height. All of a sudden this fine young man was gone.

In answer to the question: Yes, cannabis is associated with symptoms of psychosis which—for some people—can last a few hours, days, or weeks, and has been shown to trigger the early onset of certain types of psychotic disorders such as schizophrenia, whose symptoms might never go away.

How does Cannabis sometimes lead to symptoms of psychosis?

Among the approximately five-hundred chemicals found in marijuana, tetrahydrocannabinol (THC) is the chemical known to be most responsible in triggering symptoms of psychosis. Cannabis -or specifically THC- alters the functioning of parts of the brain known to be more involved in psychosis, for example it affects communication between parts of the brain called the prefrontal cortex and striatum. THC may also alter the balance of dopamine and other neurotransmitters within different parts of the brain, all of which creates a fiasco in your brain and changes the way your brain perceives reality and sensory information.

You may experience hallucinations while taking the drug (seeing things which are not there, or hearing sounds or voices which are inexistent). You may also find yourself having heightened attention or focusing on irrelevant details around you, resulting in your misinterpretation of other people's behavior (for example, thinking that people are plotting against you, are following you, or are spying on your behavior). You might also develop delusional beliefs, such as thinking that stories on the radio or television are secretly talking about you, or that the police are following or recording your every move. You might also believe yourself to be someone you're not as you disconnect more and more from reality.

Stats Corner:

- The risk of psychosis is about **3%** in the general population

- The risk of psychosis increases by **40%** for occasional cannabis users who have used it at least once in their life

- The risk of psychosis increases by **390%** for regular and heavy cannabis users [25,26,27, 41]

- Teenagers and young adults are much more at risk of psychosis when they use cannabis than adults

-Teenagers and young adults are at increased risk of falling into cannabis addiction than adults, therefore at increased risk of using cannabis regularly and consequently at increased risk of psychosis.

Again, if you're a teenager or a young adult under 25 years old, have other risk factors for developing an addiction, or have a family history of psychotic or other mental disorders, it's recommended that you avoid trying marijuana since you are at a heightened risk of developing psychotic symptoms if you try cannabis.

Why unnecessarily risk deteriorating your mental health in a way which you might never be able to reverse?

Stats corner

- Cannabis increases the risks of triggering a first episode of schizophrenia

- Cannabis may trigger symptoms of schizophrenia at an earlier age in life than would have otherwise been the case.

- 50% of people who experience a toxic psychosis (psychosis resulting from consuming drugs) will develop a chronic psychotic disorder such as schizophrenia within the next ten years.[27]

16

Cannabis - Lung Cancer

Could smoking cannabis cause lung cancer or other respiratory diseases?

"The only impossible journey is the one you never begin."
—Anthony Robins

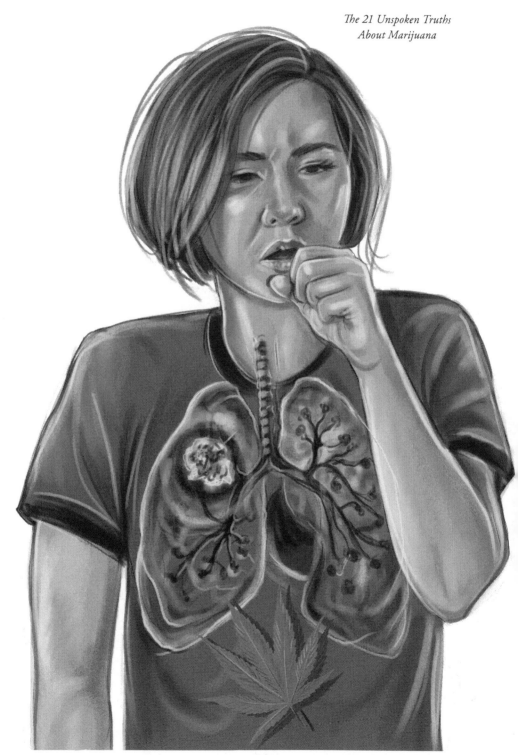

Could smoking cannabis cause lung cancer or other respiratory diseases?

Let us picture a wonderful young sixteen-year-old girl suffering from severe asthma who chooses to smoke cannabis, and thereby ends up hospitalized in the emergency room, and potentially even risking death from an exacerbated asthma attack!

Frequent and heavy marijuana smokers often have respiratory problems such as shortness of breath, and increased sputum production in their lungs due to damage to their respiratory airways… similar to the symptoms seen in heavy tobacco smokers!

It's common knowledge that smoking tobacco is associated with many kinds of cancer especially lung cancer and other respiratory diseases. According to the American Thoracic Society[28] marijuana smoke contains many of the same harmful chemicals as tobacco smoke. And for people who already have respiratory conditions such as asthma, chronic bronchitis, and emphysema, smoking marijuana could worsen these conditions in much the same ways smoking cigarettes would.

Marijuana smoke contains over 450 chemicals and a lot of cancer causing chemicals similar to tobacco smoke.[28] So if tobacco smoke is widely known to increase the risk of lung cancer, and marijuana smoke has many similar cancer causing chemicals (carcinogens), it will be very fair to conclude that Marijuana smoke increases significantly the risk of lung cancer.

17

Can Cannabis Literally Kill Someone?

"Life is like riding a bicycle. To keep your balance, you must keep moving."
—**Albert Einstein**

Marijuana overdose, not deadly, But….

This is a tough question worth considering. While almost all medical experts agree that you can't die from a marijuana overdose, the argument can be made that marijuana can kill, at least through indirect causes.

Yes, high doses of marijuana might cause an increase in heart rate which might result in increased risk of heart attack for vulnerable patients, especially those with previous heart conditions; Cannabis might cause a drop in blood pressure which may increase the risk of fainting or passing out, but these increases are usually temporary in nature. As the body gets used to the effects of marijuana these physical effects tend to decrease. While high doses of marijuana can be fatal, they are rarely directly associated with cardiac arrests, heart attacks, or strokes. Marijuana overdose therefore cannot be considered directly lethal.

> **Marijuana – cannabis - smoke might:**
>
> **- increase heart rate, which might result in increased risk of heart attack, especially for those with previous heart conditions** [42]
>
> **- increase the risk of stroke especially for the most vulnerable people with previous medical conditions**
>
> **- cause the drop of blood pressure, which might result in increased risk of fainting or passing out** [42]
>
> **- might cause damage to your blood vessels and consequently increase the risk of other associated medical conditions down the raod.**[43]

Yet a doubt still remains; what do we tell the mother of the 30-year-old man who experienced marijuana induced psychotic episodes discussed in chapter 15? This man had been fit, strong, hard-working, and wanted to enjoy life to the fullest, but since he began consuming marijuana he has been regularly hospitalized numerous times with psychotic symptoms.

This man didn't take any other drugs at all. He was doing fine, had been working on a regular basis, was considered by his friends to be a funny person, but would continually decide to start taking marijuana again, despite all the consequences he had experienced.

In search of a bigger "buzz", he smoked a little bit more than he was used to one evening, and feeling invincible, he jumped from a great height, his perception and judgment affected, and believing himself to be invincible and immortal and able to survive the jump. This lovely young man died at the scene and now he is gone forever.

Now the question is what killed him? He didn't commit suicide, and had no intention to die; he just smoked cannabis because he wanted to feel great, to enjoy life, and he didn't take any other drugs or excessive alcohol. While the week before he had been feeling great— completely normal and well-functioning—now he is gone. So what really killed him, and what is the cause of his death? It is up to the reader to answer for themselves, but one can argue that Marijuana was responsible for his death.

Can I predict how I will react to cannabis?

You cannot predict with certainty how each individual will react to taking cannabis for the first time, and it can be difficult to predict how you may react even if you've used the drug in the past. You might react fine this time, yet react badly the next time. You cannot rule out the possibility that using marijuana might lead you down the road towards feeling depressed, might trigger a psychotic episode, or could lead to dependency issues and addiction. If you are at risk of mental health problems, you may even experience psychotic or suicidal thoughts the next time you try it!

> **- You cannot know if your next experience will be like the last!**
>
> **- You can never be one-hundred percent certain how you will react, any time you take cannabis or any other drug.**

You cannot know if the next experience will be like the last. You cannot say: "I've been smoking for many years and have never had a bad experience, and never experienced a psychotic episode, so I will keep smoking and will never have a bad experience in the future". If during any particular session you increase the consumed dosage, the concentration of the product you are using happens to be stronger, or you happen to increase your frequency of use for a certain time period, you cannot predict how your brain and body might react to these changes in the amount of cannabis you put in your body....

> **Every time you put illicit drugs into your body, you are putting a certain stress on your brain, and at some point you might experience a reaction you've never experienced before. These reactions might include psychosis, anxiety, depression, suicidal thoughts or dangerously deadly behaviors.**

18

Cannabis – Car Accidents

Does cannabis increase the risk of car accidents?

"Accidents, and particularly street and highway accidents, do not happen - they are caused."
—Ernest Greenwood

The 21 Unspoken Truths About Marijuana

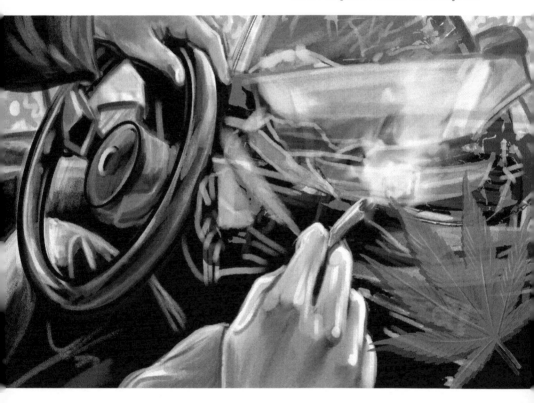

Stats Corner

- In 2016, there were 37,461 deaths from car accidents on U.S. public roads.

- In 2015, there were 1,858 Canadian deaths from car accidents.

- In 2011, there were more than 30000 deaths on European Union roads.

- A study has found a 3% increase in car accidents within U.S. states that have legalized recreational marijuana [29]

- Different studies found that drivers under marijuana influence were at least 2 times more likely to be responsible for accidents than sober drivers (drivers without alcohol, cannabis or any other drugs) [30]

Pulling out from our driveway to drive to work, to a restaurant, to visit friends, family, or someone in the hospital, our main goal is to reach our destination and to get there securely. We take all the necessary precautions to drive safely and avoid getting into an accident.

But we have no control over other drivers' actions and we are totally powerless over the way they drive! We can only hope that they will drive as safely as we do. We hope the other driver is not sleepy, is not under the influence of drugs or alcohol or intoxicated in any other way. The only control we have is to report any deviant driving to the police. And this we can do—and should do—regularly!

> - **Cannabis affects your brain and reduces attention, concentration, motor coordination, and balance.**
>
> - **These factors reduce the ability to drive safely and to react quickly to spontaneous situations which arise while driving.**[32,33]
>
> - **Therefore, cannabis significantly increases the risk of car accidents on the road not only for those who use it but for all of us on the road!**[34]

Road safety is a very distressing concern for most people. As discussed in previous chapters, cannabis use affects numerous parts of the brain such as the cerebellum (involved in balance and motor control), the basal ganglia (involved in motor control and coordination), and the prefrontal cortex (involved in focusing, paying attention, behavioral inhibition, and other crucial functions such as decision making and intuitive thinking).

In simple terms, cannabis reduces attention, concentration, motor coordination, balance, and affects reaction time. All these factors contribute in the driver's reduced ability to drive safely and to react quickly in case of abrupt or emergency circumstances on the road.

So cannabis will alter your ability to drive — as alcohol and other drugs also are known to do—and should be completely avoided if you plan to drive.

19

Does cannabis lead to suicide?

"Success is not final, failure is not fatal, it is the courage to continue that counts."
—**Winston Churchill**

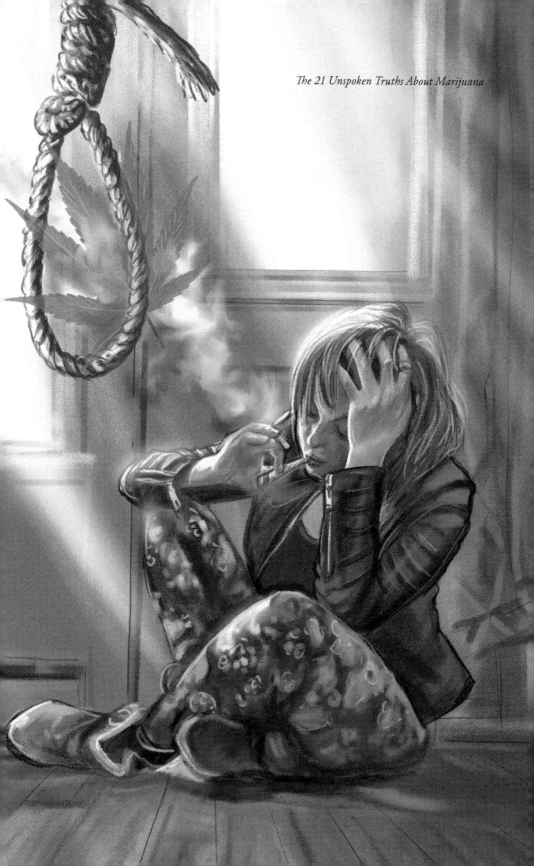

> **suicide often involves many accumulating stressful factors which put pressure on a person to the point that the problem seems irresolvable and the burden unbearable. The only way the person can envision escaping from the distress and suffering is through trying to end their life. Life still matters no matter what.**

Many factors such as physical illness, mental illness, financial stresses, bullying, divorce, academic or professional failure, social rejection, drug addiction, and sexual or physical abuse can all increase the risk of developing suicidal thoughts. There are studies which have suggested that regularly taking marijuana might also be significantly associated with increased risks of suicide (though all of these other risk factors may also play a role). But, why add yet another risk factor to your life?

This next paragraph will address the issue from another angle, but you can skip it if you're not interested in scientific theories linking cannabis use to increased risks of suicide. In down to earth terms, what happens to your brain when you take marijuana? Feelings of pleasure, euphoria, and the functioning of the brain's reward system are triggered when the brain's endocannabinoid system is activated; there are cannabinoid receptors in your brain and when you consume cannabis it binds to these receptors. However, some limited studies have produced results suggesting that people who died by suicide had a significant increase of cannabinoid receptors in some parts of the brain—especially within the prefrontal cortex—which could suggest that a hyperactive endocannabinoid system might be associated with increased risks of suicide![35,36] However, it is important to emphasize that more research is needed in this area to be able to build up more solid conclusions.

Besides having direct physiological and behavioral impacts, we know that addictions to cannabis and other substances often point to signs of other emotional problems that we could be dealing with in potentially healthier ways. We might turn to pot to try to solve our search to define our personal identity, our desire to feel we belong somewhere, as an attempt to treat or medicate our symptoms of anxiety, as an attempt to suppress our painful feelings, to put forward a mask enabling us to seem happy and functional in social situations, or as an easy way to generate pleasurable feelings instead of utilizing more meaningful sources of pleasure. Suffering is always somehow present underneath the surface contributing to seeking out marijuana, and especially so when we find ourselves using it in abusive or addictive ways instead of facing our problems head-on.

Cannabis usage—especially when it slides into addiction—might be a mask we wear to cover the profound insecurity and the profound suffering and pain.

But the more you indulge, the worse the pain, and the worse the pain, the more you indulge to soothe yourself. A cycle of personal negligence, lack of motivation, professional failure, and depression is triggered, leading you down the path towards hopelessness and potential suicidality. Still this tragic story can be avoided!!

---

*As you prepare to dive into the last chapter of this book, I suggest that you take a brief moment to explore whether you have seized all the 21 unspoken truths about marijuana discussed in this book.

Have you found the links between Marijuana/Cannabis and:		
Psychosis/schizophrenia	Depression	Anxiety
Suicide	Sleep problems	Medical uses
Car accidents	Amotivational syndrome	Social and family problems
Cognitive dysfunction	Loss of I.Q. points or ↓ intelligence	Professional and school failure
Lung cancer & Pulmonary diseases	Blood vessel damage and heart problems	Brain volume
Addiction risk	↑ Vulnerability for adolescents and young adults	Gateway drug or Front-door drug
Sex life and attachment	Second hand smoke	Pregnancy and breastfeeding

20

Proclaim Your Freedom, Reclaim Your Power!

"If you can't fly, then run. If you can't run, then walk. If you can't walk, then crawl. But by all means, keep moving."
— **Martin Luther King Jr**

You feel like your freedom has been lost, and without realizing it, cannabis has taken over your life, your family relationships, and your friendships. Your previous ambitions and personal dreams now seem unreachable. And you might be wondering how you can reclaim your power, how you can free yourself from addiction, and how you can become independent once more.

"It might not be you, it might be someone you know, someone who is dear to you who is going through a period of loss of control over drug use or other addiction. You have a desire to help and you are wondering how to proceed."

> **You might be wondering how to free yourself from dependence and become independent once more. The point is to choose your own personal path towards your freedom, and to go for it!**

There is no straight path to conquering marijuana addiction (or any other addiction for that matter). Some people turn to self-help groups, others seek help from their doctors or psychotherapists, others participate in social, physical, or recreational clubs and activities, others join churches to try to rebuild their faith after having tried every other option. The point is to choose your own personal path to reclaim your freedom, and to go for it!

Here are five simple, yet challenging suggestions; why not give them a try, knowing that you can't succeed unless you start with one step at a time!

1. YOUR PROMISE, YOUR WORDS, YOUR FREEDOM

> - **Never cease to seed beautiful words in the garden of your mind.**
>
> - **Use your mouth for you and not against you.**

At the beginning of what will realistically be a long battle, proclaim your freedom! The journey is not going to be easy, the battlefield might be harsh and cruel, but it's crucial to stay committed to staying on the frontlines. Dare to shout your commitment to becoming free; free indeed, free at last! Don't be afraid to proclaim to yourself—and to those closest to you—that you are taking responsibility towards concrete actions which will eventually result in your liberty. You are choosing to be free. Proclaim it over and over and over again!

Don't be afraid to sing, shout, and repeat how free you are in the process of becoming. Let it sink into your mind, let it penetrate your soul; you have to create your freedom in your thoughts, words, and actions. Proclaim it loud and clear!

Your thoughts and words help create reality more than you can imagine. The way you think and speak about your experience of the world helps generate conflicts and the resolutions to conflict, apprehension and anxieties, or your confidence in your successes to come. Your words can create joy or sadness, and can either help build or destroy relationships. And of course, the way you use self-talk can help build up—or destroy— the vision and reality of who you feel yourself to be, and who you are to become in the world.

> - **Choose to use your mouth to build yourself up, not to tear yourself down!**
>
> - **Stop planting negative weeds, start planting flowers**
>
> - **stop planting despair, start seeding hope!**
>
> - **Stop planting the past, start seeding the future**
>
> - **Stop planting regrets, start planting contentedness**

Proclaim your victory immediately; don't be too shy to say "I'm a winner", and to voice the intention that you are on the right track. Every victory starts in your mind, before materializing in real life. Repeat this mantra as often as you can! Be dramatic about declaring how free you're becoming! Your thoughts and words about yourself—good or bad—are infinitely more powerful than the words coming out of anyone else's mouth. Your self-talk can either give you momentum, or they can stop you in your tracks. So be conscious about the thoughts and words you are putting into the world, and be careful with them, since they can have a lasting impact on the direction your life will be taking next!

- The only way you can create a habit of speaking good things into your own life, a habit of positive self-talk, is by doing just that over and over and over again, even when you don't feel like it.

- Remember every victory starts in your mind, before materializing in real life.

---

2. GET HELP, WHEREVER YOU CAN FIND IT!

Get all the help you can, whenever you can, wherever you possibly can. Seek out all the support resources you have access to wherever you can find them, and as often as you possibly can. Whether it's through an in-patient rehab, out-patient rehabilitation center, self-help support group (for example, through Alcoholics' or Narcotics' anonymous), or church, there are numerous places we can go to, do not feel alone, dare to ask for help, search until you find. Try asking your doctor about available treatment options, go see an individual or group therapist, speak with your pastor, your priest, your religious leader, your life coach, your gym coach, your friends, your family, and see what feels right for you! Remember, you can't find what works for you if you aren't actively seeking out solutions. Again Search until you find.

You never know who will be able to steer you in the direction which will ultimately work best for you… whether it's a health professional, support group member, doctor, therapist, friend, pastor, priest, or family member that helps you make the right moves, at the right time, remain open to new ways of getting help, and don't ever give up!

> - **Don't be intimidated by your past,**
>
> - **don't let shame about your past dictate your future,**
>
> - **Don't be humiliated by failures you might have along the way**
>
> - **Just remain willing to get up every time you fall, despite the challenges, and forever committed to turning each and every failure into a learning opportunity for eventual success!**

Don't be satisfied with the status quo; search actively for answers, keep on standing up when you fall, don't wallow in feelings of shame, self-doubt, or self-pity! Remain willing to continue the fight and to go on, despite any challenge you might be facing.

Just remember that each day that passes by without you making efforts towards change means you'll be one day deeper into the problem. But once you've resolved to get help, forget about the comments naysaying friends or relatives who have negative things to say; you are investing in your life, and investing in your future. You are planting the seeds of change in your garden, and no one can take that away from you if you don't let them!

3.   U-TURN, REVERSE, DELETE!

If your life is heading in the wrong direction, it's very hard to imagine how you will ever reach your intended destination. Realistically, it may take a drastic U-turn, a change in the right direction to be able to get there. Do you know what might that change look like?

Do you need to consider putting distance between yourself and those friends who are constantly pulling you down? Don't be shy to shy away from that social group who made it so easy to make unhealthy decisions; don't hesitate to delete them from your social media contacts, don't worry about erasing their names and numbers from your phone, and getting rid of your drug dealer's information. Don't hesitate to delete, delete and delete. Don't let yourself have regrets; sometimes we need to make difficult choices to reclaim our freedom.

> **surround yourself with eagles that will help you fly,**
>
> **don't be shy to shy away from those who pull you down**

4.   NEW DISCIPLINE, NEW ROUTINE!

Build yourself a new routine and stick to it. Start eating healthy meals, and be determined to prepare food on regular schedule. Go to bed at a decent hour, and get up early with the rising sun! Start engaging in physical activities four to five times a week, and progressively start integrating more leisure and social activities in which there taking drugs isn't the primary focus.

Let's be clear: this is not going to be easy, it's actually going to be very challenging, but remember you're on the battlefield and it's not time to quit! Look for inspirational books, quotes, and advice that can keep you developing new habits of discipline, and learn to lean on your new healthier routines to stay strong and maintain your will-power in the face of hardships!

5.   ENJOY THE "NEW YOU"!

This step is all about learning to live and enjoy your life, now that you've achieved sobriety. Cannabis or other drugs produces intense and quick pleasure, so it is not going to be ease to enjoy regular drug-free leisure activities, it is going to be a learning process. Don't hesitate to learn to enjoy again, it's by walking that we learned to walk. Don't hesitate to share how far you've come in a positive and encouraging way, and to let others know how great it feels to be free again! Try not to spend time dwelling on past regrets; instead spend more time shaping your present, and creating your future. Your new routine will be instrumental in learning new ways to enjoy your new life; meet new friends, get to know new acquaintances, explore and experiment with new drug-free leisure activities, and how the whole new you experience them!

> **- It is not going to be easy to enjoy regular drug-free leisure activities, it is going to be a challenging learning process. Don't hesitate to learn to enjoy again,**
>
> **- Remember, it's by walking and falling and walking again that we all learned to walk.**
>
> **- Dare to shout your commitment to becoming free; free indeed, free at last.**

References

(1) Freeman, A. (2017, April 13). Canada announces plans to legalize marijuana by July 2018. *The Washington Post*. Retrieved from https:// www.washingtonpost.com/news/worldviews/wp/2017/04/13/ canada-announces-plans-to-legalize-marijuana-by-july-2018/

(2) Center for Behavioral Health Statistics and Quality. (2016). *2015 National Survey on Drug Use and Health: Detailed Tables*. Substance Abuse and Mental Health Services Administration, Rockville, MD. Retrieved from https://www.samhsa. gov/data/sites/default/files/NSDUH-DetTabs-2015/NSDUH-DetTabs-2015/ NSDUH-DetTabs-2015.pdf

(3) Leggett, T. (2006). A review of the world cannabis situation. *Bull Narc, 58*(1-2), 1-155.

(4) United Nations Office on Drugs and Crime. (2014). *World drug report 2014*. Retrieved from https://www.unodc.org/documents/wdr2014/ World_Drug_Report_2014_web.pdf

(5) Statistics Canada. (2015). *Canadian Tobacco, Alcohol and Drugs Survey (CTADS) 2015 summary*. Retrieved from https://www.canada.ca/en/health-canada/ services/canadian-tobacco-alcohol-drugs-survey/2015-summary.html

(6) ER Visits for Kids Rise Significantly After Pot Legalized in Colorado (2017, May 5th), *NBC News*. Retrieved from https://www.nbcnews.com/health/health-news/ er-visits-kids-rise-significantly-after-pot-legalized-colorado-n754781

(7) Center for Behavioral Health Statistics and Quality. (2013) *Drug Abuse Warning Network, 2011: National Estimates of Drug-Related Emergency Department Visits*. Substance Abuse and Mental Health Services Administration, Rockville, MD. Retrieved from https://www.samhsa.gov/data/sites/default/files/ DAWN2k11ED/DAWN2k11ED/DAWN2k11ED.pdf

(8) Steinmetz, K. (2017, April 20th). 420 Day: Why There Are So Many Different Names for Weed. *Time Magazine*. Retrieved from http://time. com/4747501/420-day-weed-marijuana-pot-slang/

(9) George, T., & Vaccarino, F. (Eds.). (2015). *Substance abuse in Canada: The Effects of Cannabis Use during Adolescence*. Ottawa, ON: Canadian Centre on

Substance Abuse. Retrieved from http://www.ccsa.ca/Resource%20Library/CCSA-Effects-of-Cannabis-Use-during-Adolescence-Report-2015-en.pdf

(10) Anthony, J. C., Warner, L. A., & Kessler, R. C. (1994). Comparative epidemiology of dependence on tobacco, alcohol, controlled substances, and inhalants: Basic findings from the national comorbidity survey. *Experimental and Clinical Psychopharmacology, 2*(3), 244.

(11) Lopez-Quintero, C., de los Cobos, José Pérez, Hasin, D. S., Okuda, M., Wang, S., Grant, B. F., & Blanco, C. (2011). Probability and predictors of transition from first use to dependence on nicotine, alcohol, cannabis, and cocaine: Results of the national epidemiologic survey on alcohol and related conditions (NESARC). *Drug and Alcohol Dependence, 115*(1), 120-130.

(12) Anthony, J.C. (2006). The epidemiology of cannabis dependence. *Cannabis Dependence: Its Nature, Consequences and Treatment.* Cambridge, UK: Cambridge University Press. 58-105.

(13) Committee opinion no. 637: Marijuana use during pregnancy and lactation. (2015). *Obstetrics & Gynecology, 126*(1), 234-238. Retrieved from https://journals.lww.com/greenjournal/Fulltext/2015/07000/Committee_Opinion_No_637_Marijuana_Use_During.48.aspx

(14) Metz, T. D., & Stickrath, E. H. (2015). Marijuana use in pregnancy and lactation: A review of the evidence. *American Journal of Obstetrics and Gynecology, 213*(6), 761-778.

(15) Goldschmidt, L., Richardson, G. A., Willford, J. A., Severtson, S. G., & Day, N. L. (2012). School achievement in 14-year-old youths prenatally exposed to marijuana. *Neurotoxicology and Teratology, 34*(1), 161-167.

(16) Goldschmidt, L., Richardson, G. A., Willford, J., & Day, N. L. (2008). Prenatal marijuana exposure and intelligence test performance at age 6. *Journal of the American Academy of Child & Adolescent Psychiatry, 47*(3), 254-263.

(17) Volkow, N. D., Wang, G., Fowler, J. S., & Tomasi, D. (2012). Addiction circuitry in the human brain. *Annual Review of Pharmacology and Toxicology, 52*, 321-336.

(18) Merline, A., Jager, J., & Schulenberg, J. E. (2008). Adolescent risk factors for adult alcohol use and abuse: Stability and change of predictive value across early and middle adulthood. *Addiction, 103*(s1), 84-99.

(19) Zimmermann, P., Wittchen, H., Waszak, F., Nocon, A., Höfler, M., & Lieb, R. (2005). Pathways into ecstasy use: The role of prior cannabis use and ecstasy availability. *Drug and Alcohol Dependence, 79*(3), 331-341.

(20) NIDA. (2018). Marijuana. Retrieved from https://www.drugabuse.gov/drugs-abuse/marijuana on January 19, 2018

(21) Weinberger, A. H., Platt, J., & Goodwin, R. D. (2016). Is cannabis use associated with an increased risk of onset and persistence of alcohol use disorders? A three-year prospective study among adults in the united states. *Drug and Alcohol Dependence, 161*, 363-367.

(22) Meier, M. H., Caspi, A., Ambler, A., Harrington, H., Houts, R., Keefe, R. S., . . . Moffitt, T. E. (2012). Persistent cannabis users show neuropsychological decline from childhood to midlife. *Proceedings of the National Academy of Sciences of the United States of America, 109*(40), E2657-64. doi:10.1073/pnas.1206820109 [doi].

(23) Center for Behavioral Health Statistics and Quality. (2013) *Drug Abuse Warning Network, 2011: National Estimates of Drug-Related Emergency Department Visits.* Substance Abuse and Mental Health Services Administration, Rockville, MD. Retrieved from https://www.samhsa.gov/data/sites/default/files/DAWN2k11ED/DAWN2k11ED/DAWN2k11ED.pdf

(24) Degenhardt, L., Chiu, W., Sampson, N., Kessler, R. C., Anthony, J. C., Angermeyer, M., . . . Huang, Y. (2008). Toward a global view of alcohol, tobacco, cannabis, and cocaine use: Findings from the WHO world mental health surveys. *PLoS Medicine, 5*(7), e141.

(25) Moore, T. H., Zammit, S., Lingford-Hughes, A., Barnes, T. R., Jones, P. B., Burke, M., & Lewis, G. (2007). Cannabis use and risk of psychotic or affective mental health outcomes: A systematic review. *The Lancet, 370*(9584), 319-328.

(26) Grant, C. N., & Bélanger, R. E. (2017). Cannabis and Canada's children and youth. *Paediatrics & Child Health, 22*(2), 98-102.

(27) Arendt, M., Rosenberg, R., Foldager, L., Perto, G., & Munk-Jorgensen, P. (2005). Cannabis-induced psychosis and subsequent schizophrenia-spectrum disorders: Follow-up study of 535 incident cases. *The British Journal of Psychiatry : The Journal of Mental Science, 187,* 510-515. doi:187/6/510 [pii]

(28) American Thoracic Society. (2017). *Smoking marijuana and the lungs.* Retrieved from https://www.thoracic.org/patients/patient-resources/resources/marijuana.pdf

(29) Leefeldt, E. (2017, June 22). Legal pot and car crashes: Yes, there's a link. *CBS News.* Retrieved from https://www.cbsnews.com/news/legal-pot-and-car-crashes-yes-theres-a-link/

(30) Elvik, R. (2013). Risk of road accident associated with the use of drugs: A systematic review and meta-analysis of evidence from epidemiological studies. *Accident Analysis & Prevention, 60,* 254-267.

(31) Center for Behavioral Health Statistics and Quality. (2013) *Drug Abuse Warning Network, 2011: National Estimates of Drug-Related Emergency Department Visits.* Substance Abuse and Mental Health Services Administration, Rockville, MD. Retrieved from https://www.samhsa.gov/data/sites/default/files/DAWN2k11ED/DAWN2k11ED/DAWN2k11ED.pdf

(32) Lenné, M. G., Dietze, P. M., Triggs, T. J., Walmsley, S., Murphy, B., & Redman, J. R. (2010). The effects of cannabis and alcohol on simulated arterial driving: Influences of driving experience and task demand. *Accident Analysis & Prevention, 42*(3), 859-866.

(33) Hartman, R. L., & Huestis, M. A. (2013). Cannabis effects on driving skills. *Clinical Chemistry, 59*(3), 478-492. doi:10.1373/clinchem.2012.194381 [doi]

(34) Asbridge, M., Poulin, C., & Donato, A. (2005). Motor vehicle collision risk and driving under the influence of cannabis: Evidence from adolescents in atlantic canada. *Accident Analysis & Prevention, 37*(6), 1025-1034. Retrieved from http://www.bmj.com/content/bmj/344/bmj.e536.full.pdf

(35) Dwivedi, Y. (2012). *The Neurobiological Basis of Suicide.* Boca Raton (FL): CRC Press/Taylor & Francis. Retrieved from https://www.ncbi.nlm.nih.gov/books/NBK107200/

(36) Serra, G., & Fratta, W. (2007). A possible role for the endocannabinoid system in the neurobiology of depression. *Clinical Practice and Epidemiology in Mental Health, 3*(1), 25.

(37) Asbridge, M., Poulin, C., & Donato, A. (2005). Motor vehicle collision risk and driving under the influence of cannabis: Evidence from adolescents in atlantic canada. *Accident Analysis & Prevention, 37*(6), 1025-1034.

(38) Carliner, H., Mauro, P. M., Brown, Q. L., Shmulewitz, D., Rahim-Juwel, R., Sarvet, A. L., . . . Hasin, D. S. (2017). The widening gender gap in marijuana use prevalence in the US during a period of economic change, 2002–2014. *Drug and Alcohol Dependence, 170*, 51-58.

(39) Rubino, T., Zamberletti, E., & Parolaro, D. (2012). Adolescent exposure to cannabis as a risk factor for psychiatric disorders. *Journal of Psychopharmacology, 26*(1), 177-188.

(40) Rey, J. M., Sawyer, M. G., Raphael, B., Patton, G. C., & Lynskey, M. (2002). Mental health of teenagers who use cannabis. results of an australian survey. *The British Journal of Psychiatry : The Journal of Mental Science, 180*, 216-221.

(41) Association des Médecins Psychiatres du Québec (AMPQ). *Legalization of Cannabis: Let's protect Future Generations.* position paper (2017, June 3). Retrieved from http://ampq.org/wp-content/uploads/2017/06/enonce-de-positionanglais1.pdf

(42) Thomas et al. (2014). Adverse cardiovascular, cerebrovascular, and peripheral vascular effects of marijuana inhalation: what cardiologists need to know. American Journal of Cardiology 113(1): 187–90. http://www.ajconline.org/article/S0002-9149(13)01976-0/fulltext

(43) Wang et al. (2016). One minute of marijuana secondhand smoke exposure substantially impairs vascular endothelial function. Journal of the American Heart Association. 5(8). https://www.ncbi.nlm.nih.gov/pmc/articles/PMC5015303/

Made in the USA
Columbia, SC
31 August 2018